A Weighty Issue

By
Lynne D M Noble

Copyright 2018 Lynne D M Noble

This book shall not, by way of trade or otherwise, be lent, re-sold, hired out, or otherwise circulated without the prior consent of the copyright holder or the publisher in any form of binding or cover than that in which it is published and without a similar condition including this condition being imposed on the subsequent purchaser.
 The use of its contents in another media is also subject to the same conditions.

Independently published

Acknowledgement

To all those who inspired me to write this book by sharing their stories with me

About the Author

Lynne Noble was born in 1953 in Huddersfield, West Yorkshire. From a very early age, Lynne showed an interest in nutrition and genetics avidly reading any books that she could get her hands on at the time.

Initially, Lynne studied orthopaedics but events led her to work with the elderly mentally infirm. Here, her interest in neurodegenerative disorders and pain syndromes developed.

Lynne undertook rigorous programmes of study, completing her Cert Ed., (FE) BSc (Hons) and Adv. Dip Education simultaneously before moving onto her M.Ed.

From there she took further demanding programmes in Human Nutrition, Pharmacology, Neuroscience, Genetics and Immunology. During this time, she was given many prestigious awards for her academic work. It was noted then that Lynne was not afraid of tackling difficult subjects.

She began her law degree but ill health prevented her from pursuing this. However, in this time, she moved from being a foster parent to adoptive parent.

She has been instrumental in setting up projects in the community for disadvantaged groups.

She is a member of the Guild of Health Writers and the British Union of Journalists.

Now retired, she lives in a picturesque village in West Yorkshire with her husband. She enjoys gardening, watching her husband bowling and researching.

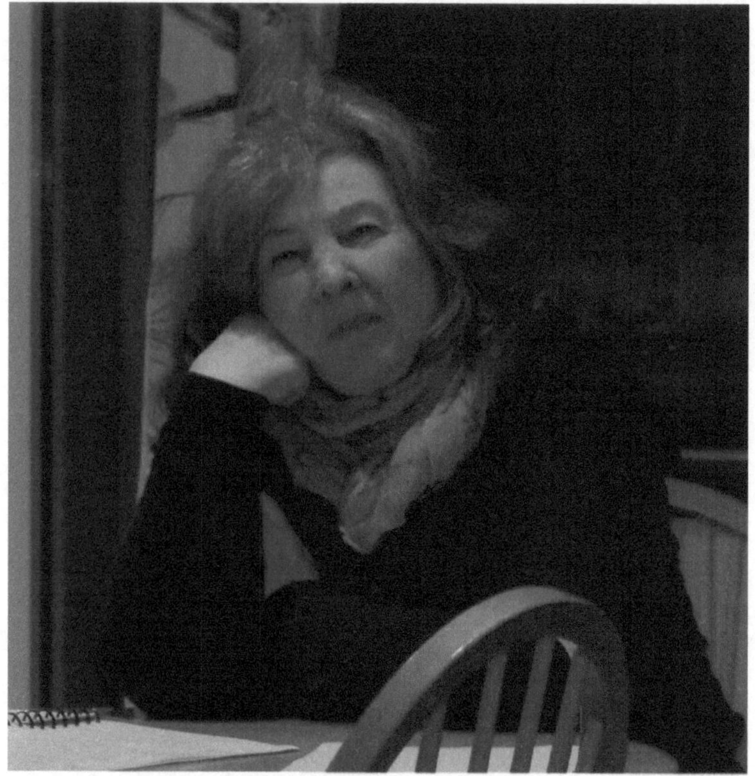

Author Lynne Noble at home

https://quintessentiallylynne.weebly.com/nutritional-medicine.html

Contents

Preface

The issue of body weight continues to be a major topic of conversation in our society. Our personality traits are judged by how much we weigh, our health is determined by where we fall on the Body Mass Index and we judge ourselves on how loveable we are depending on our body mass.

Our scales appear unforgiving. We are convinced they are wrong or need oiling or replacing. We find that if we lean forward a little when standing on the weighing scales that this will reduce our weight by half a pound. This cheers us up and so our view of life and how we measure up is determined by a small object standing in the corner of the bathroom.

We are constantly informed that if our body mass index rises above a certain amount then we will be considered obese. Up to that point we have felt fine. We hold down a job, we are popular with friends and family, we look good in the clothes we have bought and we feel healthy. Now, we are being informed that we are increasing the risk factors for heart disease and stroke, arthritis and high blood pressure. We recall Aunt Joan who would have been deemed obese by the Body Mass Index. She lived until she was 102 years of age. Up until three months before she died, she did all her own washing and housework and had never had so much as a cold never mind a heart attack or stroke. Perhaps if she hadn't been 'obese' she might have lived until she was 108. Who knows?

Sometimes we can have very unrealistic expectations about our body size. I recall an acquaintance, who was in her thirties, stating that she didn't look like she did when she was fifteen and wanted her fifteen old shape back again as her husband preferred her like that. I think in this case that it was the husband who had a problem. Fifteen-year old girls are not fully developed and further physical maturing will occur. However, it does demonstrate how easily we can be influenced into not loving ourselves, by others.

Perceptions of the ideal body shape does change over time. In the early 1900's, the idea of a beautiful body was influenced by Charles Dana Gibson who portrayed the ideal figure for a woman as being tall with a slender waist but having a voluptuous bosom, hips and buttocks. However, women did not naturally have this shape, they achieved their S-curved torso by using an uncomfortable swan bill corset.

Curves became more fashionable in the 1930's to 1940's.

In the 1960's Twiggy (Lesley Lawson) dominated the fashion scene. She was well known for her thin, boyish build, short hair and her big eyes enhanced by long eyelashes.

The shift dress was fashionable at the time and suited this shape perfectly. Curves were out and mini- skirts were in. Teenagers spent hours using eyeliner to achieve the 'look' which was all the rage. In many a sense, this fashion suited those entering their teens since they had not developed physically and attained the fuller curves, which develop later. Breasts and curvaceous hips were hankered for as a sign of their blossoming adulthood. This was wrapped up in their 'right' to a newer and greater freedom.

The intense emotion which often occurs alongside puberty will be associated with the fashion of the time; it is part of that we use to establish our identity. As we get older, people often find themselves hankering after the 'good old days' and harking back to when life was relatively freer and with less responsibility than it has now. Association is indeed powerful.

However, we can see how we yearn for what we don't have. The teens desire physical evidence of their passage into adult hood and those who have left their teens behind desire the look of the slim hipped boyishness of their teens.

Since Twiggy we have had various other fashion leaders who influence how we feel about ourselves. Kate Moss, in the 1990's introduced the 'waif' like appearance to the catwalk. More recently, Kim Kardashian and Beyonce have 'legitimised' large buttocks.

How we feel about ourselves can very much depend on the era we were brought up in. Taking this a little further though, we do not have to blindly follow another's fashion ideal, we could learn to make fashion. In other words, by confidently establishing what our basic body features are we can create the next fashion just as Charles Dana Gibson did with his Gibson girls drawing. We do have the choice whether to define any feature positively or negatively. If we wish to accentuate our breasts we have push up balcony bras. Alternatively, if we wish to minimise them then there are bras that distribute breast tissue so that the size is not so pronounced.

However, our figures have *generally* undergone marked changes over the past couple of decades. There are a number of reasons which could account for this. We have a wider range of food to choose from. It is easily available so we don't have to expend too much energy in getting it. We have more disposable income at our fingertips and so can buy more than we need. We generally exercise less. We can understand, in some part, how these changes have happened.

For some people though, their body mass probably isn't healthy or they want to feel better about themselves. They want to be able to feel comfortable wearing something different. Their weight has crept up and they don't know why. They feel less healthy or less confident because of it. They can tell you all about the latest diet fads - and, indeed, will have tried most of them out – but they cannot shift those few extra pounds.

There are a number of well recognised life events when weight is likely to rise and these include such events as post pregnancy, times of stress and mid-life. Why weight gain or size differences are likely to occur at these various times often differs. It is not always about the amount of calories taken in, being more than the amount of calories expended.

This book addresses a number of problems for those who have gained unwanted weight – and are finding it difficult to lose - or found that their dress size has increased against their will or understanding. It will also explore whether obesity is as unhealthy as it is said to be or whether obesity has some advantages over those who are deemed non-obese.   Many of the insights provided in this book are unlikely to be found in other books of a similar nature. It is a unique guide to some of the weightier issues in life, why they might occur and how to address them.

The BMI Index is Useless

When people attend their General Practitioner then one of the measurements taken at the time is body mass. This is then plotted on a chart and the results are channelled into a bald statement which determine whether you are

- Underweight
- Normal weight
- Obese
- Morbidly Obese

The Body Mass Index (BMI) is not an accurate measure of fat. It doesn't explain the causes of poor health.

In some cases, obesity can be a risk factor for diabetes, heart disease and death but only in those with a genetic propensity to such illnesses. In many cases obesity actually increases survival time in those with chronic illness. Therefore, individuals with a high BMI with chronic illness such as heart failure or kidney failure, among others, are more likely to have increased survival rates. It is thought that having more fat provides additional energy reserves.

The guidelines set by the World Health Organisation (WHO) stated that a BMI of over 25 is considered to be overweight while a BMI of more than 30 would indicate that the individual is obese. However, this criterion fails to take into consideration a number of groups for which such criterion would fail to apply.

The criterion fails to address large number of people in Asia such as Japanese and Koreans. They experienced metabolic risks, such as diabetes and hypertension, at a much lower threshold. Even with a BMI of 23 or 24, studies found that a significant number of people of Japanese or Korean descent had those diseases.

Studies also show that the current BMI recommendations are not suitable for older adults.

A study undertaken by Caryl Nowson, who was a professor of nutrition and aging at Deakin University, examined the relationship between BMI and risk of death in people 65 and over.

The findings indicated that there was a lower risk of death in those with a BMI which fell into the obese category. Further, it was found that mortality increased significantly among those with a BMI in the 'normal' weight range. Further studies found that those with BMI in the obese range had a reduced risk of dying compared to those whose BMI was 21 or 22 – that is, in the normal range. The findings were that, 'by current standards, being overweight is not associated with an increased risk of dying.

Professor Nowson stated

Rather it is those sitting at the lower end of the normal range that need to be monitored, as older people with BMI's less than 23 are at an increased risk of dying.'

He added

Rather than focussing on weight loss, older people should put their efforts into having a balanced diet, eating when hungry and keeping active.'

Some studies have demonstrated that some obese individuals have a lower cardiovascular risk while many individuals with a normal BMI are metabolically unhealthy and have an increased mortality risk.

Obesity is not always associated with joint problems. Inflammation is generally associated with joint problems and this is more of a concern of nutritional intake rather than obesity. Of course with any medical condition some individuals have more of a propensity to such conditions, than others. That means they will have to pay more attention to their diets than those not predisposed to joint problems.[1]

Obese people have better post-surgical short-term survival rates among obese people than patients of 'normal' weight.' Patients with a BMI of 23.1 or less were more than twice as likely to die within 30 days of surgery than those with a BMI of 35.5 or more.

---

[1] Glycine and phenylalanine, chondroitin and glucosamine are nutrients which assist in good joint health.

The BMI also exaggerates thinness in short people and fatness in tall people. Further, it does not take into account the person's body fat versus muscle (lean tissue). As such it is a very flawed measure of a person's body fat.

It is not worth the paper it is printed on since it was devised for an entirely different purpose.

Exercise can help in losing weight for a number of reasons

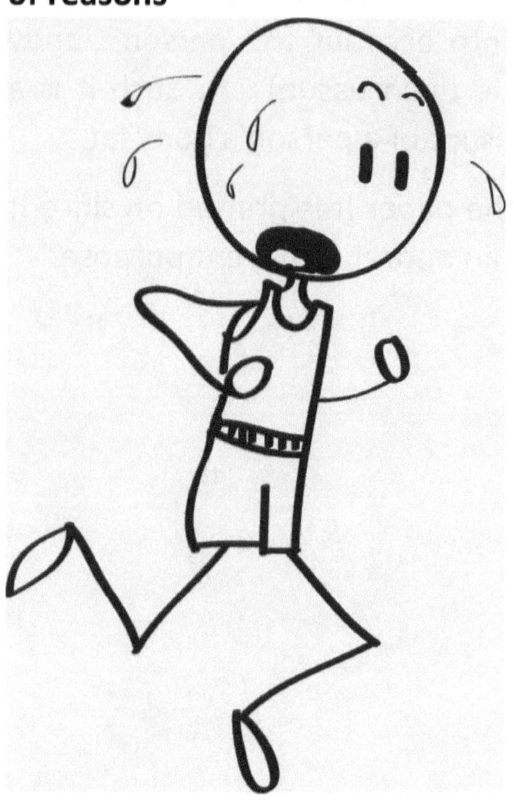

When we think of exercise, it is not generally in the context of a gentle stroll down to the shops or the effort involved in doing the housework such as making the beds or pushing the vacuum cleaner. Exercise is normally thought of in the context of a brisk hill walking or lifting weights. They can help with losing weight - although in the case of weight lifting it is more likely to increase weight - but, for most people, such exercise is not a palatable thought and not many people have time to spend hours walking in the hills.

The reason why weight lifting can increase weight is that it builds muscle. Muscle weighs more than fat. However, such exercise can help define and tone necessitating a smaller size in clothing even if weight loss does not occur.

Exercise does burn calories. Energy has to be released in order for it to power muscles. However, exercise, in some unfortunates, can induce hunger. In the short term it does with me.

In the longer term I find it is an appetite suppressant.

 The difficulty is that I do far more short bursts of exercise than I ever do extended bouts. At such times I am far more likely to take in more calories through eating a snack, than I ever am likely to expend energy on exercise.

I don't snack on fruit. I never have done. I generally feel quite light headed after eating a piece of fruit - a phenomenon I associate with potassium's ability to lower blood pressure.

 Fruit is a good source of potassium.

When I look at the amount of calories I expend in 15 minutes of moderate walking to the local shops, I find it is only a modest 36 calories. If I allow for the return journey, then I have used a total of 72 calories. Walking briskly does increase the amount of calories burned but not by much. An average chocolate bar contains about 250 calories.

Walking to the shops after a meal has obvious advantages in that you will have plenty of available energy. Further studies show that individuals spend less when they are not hungry.

Why does physical exercise have the potential to create hunger?

Whenever the body is under a state of stress, it releases cortisol. Cortisol is the anti-stress hormone and when it is released into the bloodstream it can act on many different parts of the body and help it to respond to stress or danger.

 Cortisol also helps increase the body's metabolism of glucose.

Cortisol is a necessary stress hormone that is designed to aid wakefulness in the morning as

Stress can increase the risk for obesity

well as enable us to cope with danger. An increase in cortisol also triggers the release of amino acids from the muscles, fatty acids into the blood stream as well as glucose from the liver.

 This all helps us access an enormous amount of energy should we need it in an emergency.

Cortisol also stimulates insulin release and maintenance of blood sugar levels. The consequence of all the above is an increase in appetite especially in relation to sweet, high fat and salty foods.

Insulin resistance is a particular problem as it may lead to an increase in blood sugar. High blood sugar levels can cause a lot of systemic damage. We really want the blood sugar to be pushed into cells and provide fuel for cells rather than circulate in the blood. This is what provides our energy.

When insulin resistance abounds, weight gain is one of the side effects.

We can translate the effects of cortisol to other stressors in our life which have the potential to cause weight gain.

Often we have been so inculcated into thinking that our way of life is the 'norm' that we don't explore the damage that it is doing to us. Some common examples of stressors which have the potential to raise cortisol and impact weight are:

- Caffeinated drinks
- Lack of sleep
- Driving
- Light pollution

- Noise pollution
- Relationship difficulties
- Working in a less than satisfying job
- Not having enough time to do things
- Being too cold
- Being too hot
- Children
- Illness
- Injury
- Dealing with utilities and similar organisations
- Divorce
- Bereavement

Please feel free to add some of your own.

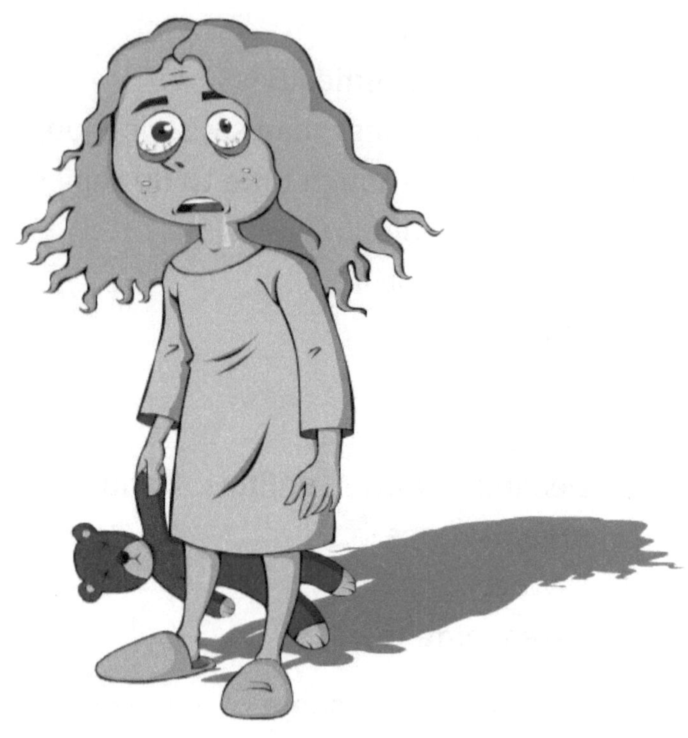

Insomnia is associated with obesity.

It is perhaps not difficult to see that the more developed our lives or countries are, the more likely we are to suffer from *unwanted* obesity that is not necessarily associated with over eating.

Extended exercise (more than 20 minutes) will use up the energy released by cortisol. It will also help to control insulin resistance so that the fuel released can be used by cells.

When cortisol levels are elevated, the body also produces less testosterone. This will result in a decrease in muscle mass.   You need testosterone to build muscle mass.

 Muscle helps to burn calories. However, a reduced muscle mass, will burn fewer calories.

Stress can also alter the normal pattern of cortisol secretion. Normally levels are highest in the morning and lowest at night. As levels of cortisol lessen, melatonin increases.

 Melatonin is a hormone which regulates the sleep wake cycle. When melatonin is disrupted by wayward cortisol levels then sleep escapes us.

 This disrupted sleep pattern causes further stress. A vicious circle begins.

This disruption of cortisol secretion doesn't just promote weight gain; it also decides where that weight gain will occur. Stress coupled with elevated cortisol will cause fat deposition in the abdominal area as opposed to the hips.

 This apple shaped abdominal obesity is unhealthy, compared to the pear shaped figure of an obese individual, where such fat deposition has not been caused by raised cortisol levels.

It is the apple shaped abdominal fat deposition which is associated with cardiovascular disease which includes stroke and heart attacks. This is a far better indicator of poor health than the BMI.

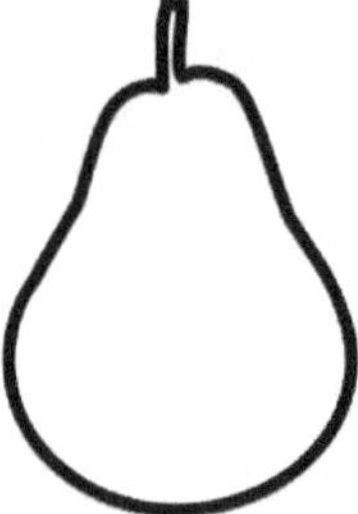 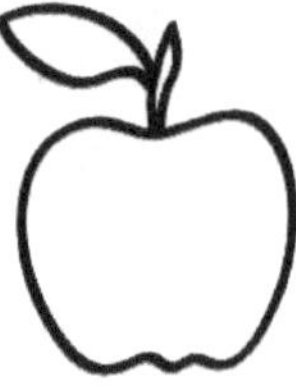

Better pear shaped than apple shaped.

 If you find that you have a tendency to an apple shape, then you need to investigate the stressors in your life and seek to eliminate them. This isn't always easy and sometimes an innovative approach has to be considered, or help sought from other quarters. For example, if money is tight then

- growing your own food or
- learning how to harvest it for free from the countryside or
- joining a cookery class which teaches you how to cook cheaper meals, can help as well as provide new friendships.

Some people love living frugally – I do – but others find it stressful.

If coffee is a stressor, then find a decaffeinated blend or try something entirely different. I am not keen on herbal teas but I don't mind the decaffeinated black teas at all.

Our bungalow is also a sun trap in the summer. The intensity of the sunlight is a major stressor for me. I found that even when I closed the curtains there was still too much blinding light getting through; it caused me major problems.

I solved this by asking an organisation to place film over the windows which keeps the majority of the very intense light out.

Other Symptoms of excessive cortisol levels are

- Weight gain around the upper back
- Rounding of the face
- Flushed face
- Thinning skin
- Easy bruising
- Muscle weakness
- Delayed healing

Exercise and the Lymphatic System

The lymphatic system runs parallel to the circulatory system. It contains hundreds of lymphatic vessels and bean shaped nodes throughout the body. It carries a clear fluid known as lymph throughout the body. This fluid helps to deliver essential white blood cells to sites of infection to fight disease

The lymph system can become clogged with dead bacteria and other waste. Unlike the circulatory system which has a pump – the heart – the lymphatic system does not. To get lymph moving you need to move. It is a slow process unclogging the lymphatic system but the consequences of this, if exercise is not undertaken, is that swelling will occur. If it is allowed to continue then infection and disease will occur.

When lymph builds up it can cause weight gain but this is due to lymph not adipose tissue.

It can also increase the need for a larger clothing size.

Lymph can be helped to move by **light** support.

Lymph has to travel against gravity so it has an uphill struggle. Tight clothing, however, does not help at all. The lymph vessels are very delicate and tight clothing will just compress them so that the lymph cannot flow. Therefore, when out walking, wear comfortable loose clothing.

Slow, relaxed breathing also helps to activate the lymph system. Our general pattern of breathing has become quicker and shallower and generally reflects the fast pace of life which is ours.

A considerable amount of weight can be lost without dieting just by attending to the needs to the lymphatic system. Dry brushing and elevating the foot of the bed is also beneficial for getting lymph to flow.

There is also a special form of light massage called lymphatic drainage which may be beneficial. However, the weight that will be lost will not be fat, it will be excess lymph fluid which can weigh a considerable amount. While fat is not lost, the excess fluid lost can result in a much more contoured shape.

A clogged lymphatic system is more likely in

- The elderly
- Those who have had a recent infection
- Those who don't exercise much

- Those who have had an injury which has damaged the fragile lymph vessels

Lymphoedema differs in that it is a chronic disease and requires much more - and ongoing -attention.

However, a poorly functioning or backed up lymphatic system can cause significant weight gain which has nothing to do with an excess of calories.

Growth Hormone and GABA

Most people have heard of Human Growth Hormone (HGH) but do not generally know what it is or what it does. This chapter will then give insight into a vitally important anti-ageing substance.

HGH is a hormone which is made in the pituitary gland. AS we age, the body's HGH levels decrease, which have led some scientists to believe that if we could raise HGH levels then this has the potential to reverse some of the effects of the ageing process. However, when HGH is taken by mouth it is destroyed in the acidic environment of the stomach. In order to benefit from HGH it has to bypass the stomach and be injected.

It is possible to purchase injectable HGH online and some GP's may prescribe it off label. However, this is not the easiest way to obtain HGH.

There are a lot of pills and potions that are sold which state either contain HGH or will help produce it in the body. Those containing HGH will not work given that they will be destroyed in the stomach so we will have to look at the products which are not destroyed in the stomach that may help produce HGH in the body.

A study showed that oral administration of an amino acid which is also an inhibitory neurotransmitter elevated resting serum growth hormone concentrations.

The purpose of the study[2] was to test the hypothesis that GABA ingestion stimulates

---

[2]

https://www.ncbi.nlm.nih.gov/pubmed/180910 16

immunoreactive GH (irGH) and immunofunctional GH(ifGH) release at rest.

Eleven resistance trained men (18-30 years) participated in this randomised, double blind, placebo-controlled, cross over study. During each experimental bout, participants ingested 3g of GABA or a placebo (P), followed either by resting or resistance exercise session. Fasting venous blood samples were taken at various intervals.

At rest the participants who'd had GABA were tested with those who had the placebo. The conclusions reached from the data were that ingested GABA elevates resting and post exercise irGH and ifGH concentrations. However, the extent to which it contributes to muscle growth is not known.

Now that we have shown that HGH can occur due to the ingestion of GABA, then it would be useful to know what we can expect if we take GABA supplements. These are:

- Loss of fat and muscle gain

- Increased energy levels
- Increased cardiac output
- Fewer wrinkles and improved skin elasticity
- Increased bone mass
- Increased memory retention
- Enhanced sexual appetite
- Improved sleep quality

GABA may also contribute to weight loss by its ability to induce restful sleep. A good night's sleep is associated with weight loss since this is when HGH is released. People who take GABA tend to lose weight quite effortlessly, this includes even the dreaded middle age spread, which afflicts many, and is difficult to get rid of. As there is loss of fat and muscle gain, the body becomes much more contoured too.

GABA is normally prescribed in doses of 200mg before bedtime to aid restful sleep. However, its fat burning capabilities, which are linked to the production of HGH, would require doses of approximately 3g on an empty stomach before bed. However, it is better to start at 1g and work up in 500mg increments daily until you find a dose which aids sleep. This dose would also promote weight loss.

In the UK, it has just become illegal to sell substances which promote HGH. This ban is indicative of the effectiveness of GABA in helping increase levels of HGH.

However, GABA can be bought online.

There aren't any foods which contain GABA. It is made from another amino acid, glutamine, which is found in animal protein such as meat, fish, eggs and cheese. However, GABA is synthesised during fermentation, so eating foods like yogurt, kimchi, kefir and cheese all help to increase GABA levels which can subsequently help to increase HGH levels.

Studies on yogurt, which showed that ingestion of it resulted in weight loss, was attributed to the calcium it contains. However, it is more likely that weight loss was as a result of the fermentation process involved, which produced GABA.

L-theanine – another amino acid has been shown to increase GABA, serotonin and dopamine. It also helps to decrease cortisol. L-theanine is rapidly absorbed and results in reduced anxiety within a few minutes.

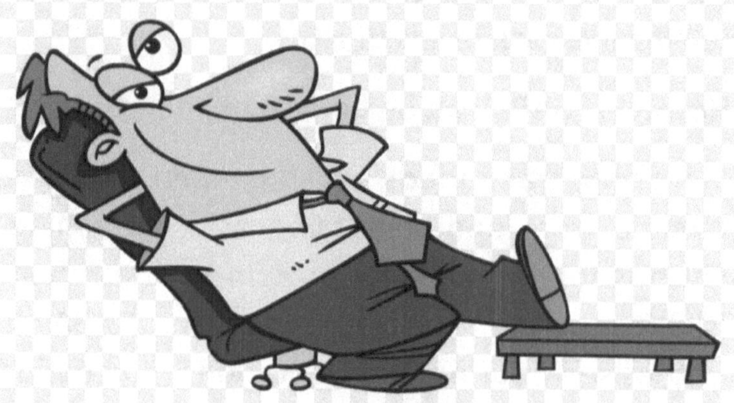

L-theanine results in reduced anxiety within minutes.

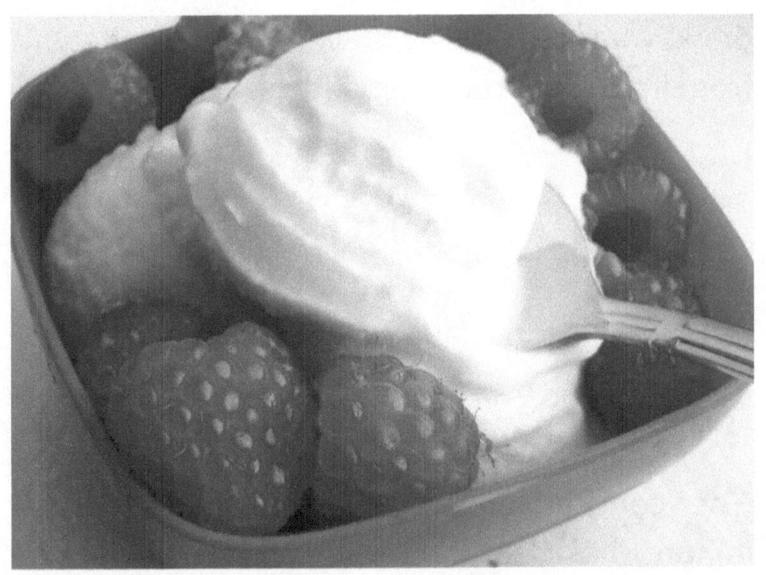

Yogurt can help increase GABA levels through its fermentation process

However, L-theanine has very few natural sources. It can be found in mushrooms but, mostly, it is found in the leaves of tea. This is why people reach for a cup of tea when they are feeling anxious and need to wind down. L-theanine really does help individuals to relax.

When tea is brewed most of the L-theanine does end up in the tea rather than remain within the leaves. Therefore, it makes sense to drink your tea strong if you want to benefit from its anxiety reducing effects.

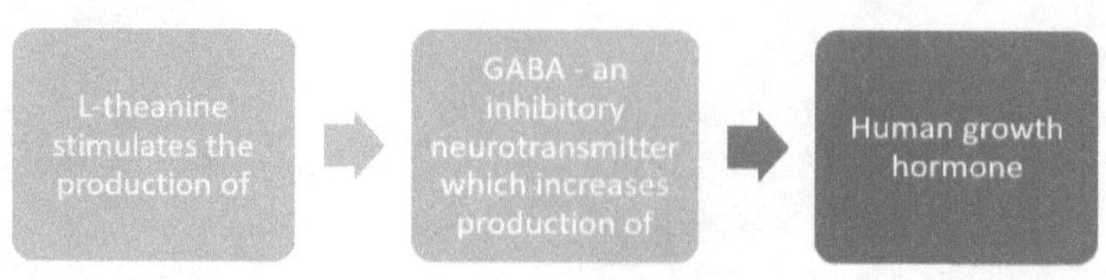

The concept of brewing the tea for three minutes has clear benefits. Leftover tea can be used in lots of ways, too. It was not unusual to soak dried fruit in cold tea before making the Christmas pudding. The Victorians really did know how to not waste anything.

Further, a couple of tablespoons of strong cold tea, incorporated into a coffee or chocolate cake, will not add such a strong flavour that it becomes unpalatable while adding to its beneficial effects on mood.

Green tea is also promoted as having properties which aid weight loss. It too, has a good amount of L-theanine in it that is able to increase the availability of GABA.

 Here is an iced green tea recipe for you to try.

Ingredients:

2 pints of water

4-6 green tea bags

One orange and one lemon sliced

Sweetening agent – honey, sugar, sweetener

Method

Place all the ingredients – apart from the fruit - in a jar with a fitted lid. Place in a warm place for 3-4 hours.

After this time add the fruit and place back in a warm place for a couple of hours.

Serve over ice after it has been sweetened further, to taste, if desired.

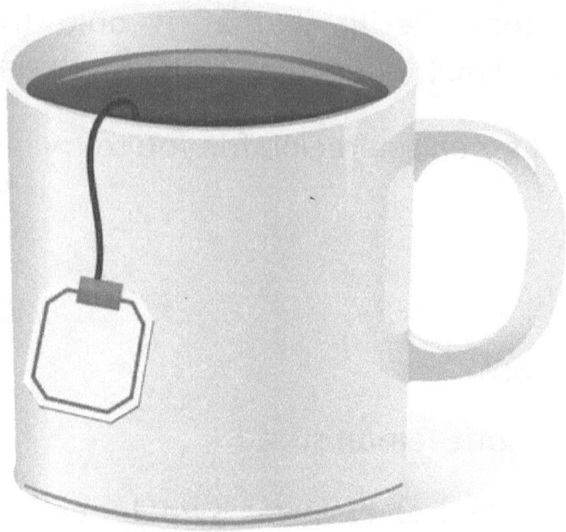

There is sound scientific reasoning why a cup of tea has 'pick me up' properties.

Some medications which cause weight gain

It is probably true to say that there are more medications which induce weight gain than there are which result in weight loss. Unfortunately, many of these are medications which are prescribed on a frequent basis.

Antihistamines are well known for causing significant weight gain. They appear to do this by inhibiting histamine. Histamine is released as an early response to injury or the presence of an allergen. It causes symptoms such as itchy, runny noses, urticaria (nettle rash) streaming eyes, among others. It can also cause achy joints and muscles in some people.

Histamine suppresses appetite so one effect of taking antihistamines is an increase in appetite. This doesn't appear to be the whole story, in our quest for causes of weight gain, since some antihistamines appear to cause more weight gain than others; currently. there does not appear to be a known explanation for this.

Studies have shown that those taking antihistamines can be up to two stone heavier than those who aren't.

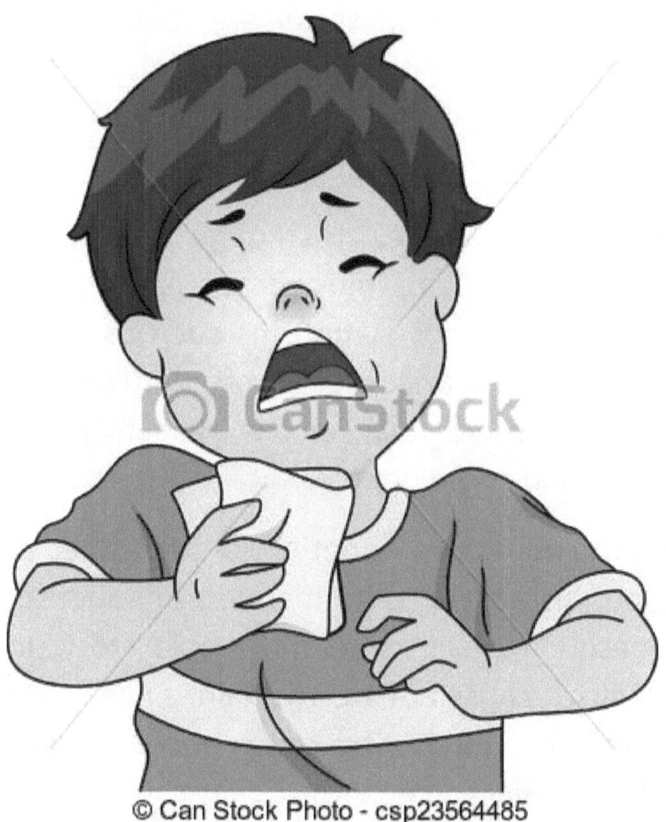

Anti-histamines are taken by people with allergies

Some high histamine foods are

- Pickled foods
- Fermented food such as sauerkraut, yogurt, sour cream, buttermilk, kefir, cheese
- Cured or fermented meats – sausages, salami and fermented ham.

If your diet is high in these foods it is quite likely that you will have unwanted weight gain.

The two main culprits of antihistamines are

- Fenofexadine
- Cetirizine

Antihistamines also have a sedating effect and it may account for less exercise being taken so that calorie expenditure is reduced.

This explanation cannot account for the whole story though. Some antacids such as Ranitidine and Omeprazole, which act on similar receptors, also cause quite marked weight gain and without the sedating effects. It may be that a reduction in symptoms which such antacids bring may increase a desire to eat. However, I am not sure that this accounts for the marked increase in weight gain that antihistamines and antacids bring. And Ranitidine has been found to cause modest weight loss in some individuals.[3]

A natural substance, quercetin, which is found in many vegetables especially those in the onion family have been found to counteract allergies but without the side effects of antihistamines.

However, by far the best natural antihistamine is vitamin C and it has the added bonus of not being associated with weight gain.

---

[3] Ranitidine has also be found to cause modest weight loss in some people.

Non-steroidal anti-inflammatory drugs (NSAID's)

NSAID's such as ibuprofen do not cause an increase in body fat, but they do cause weight gain in the form of excess water, known as oedema. Ibuprofen does not increase your appetite so any weight gain, due to excess fluid, will disappear once the medication has been stopped.

NSAID'S should not be used in those with kidney problems or those on methotrexate. In addition, NSAID's are often implicated in allergies, or anaphylaxis, for which the treatment offered is an antihistamine.

As we have seen these have the potential to cause weight gain.

Diuretics and Laxatives

These are a major cause of weight gain although most people take them in the hope that they will cause weight loss. Taking diuretics and laxatives will cause potassium loss. This state is known as hypokalaemia.

Many of the symptoms of hypokalaemia are non-specific. Weakness and fatigue are the most common complaints; the muscle weakness, which occurs, is manifested in a number of ways such as

- Shortness of breath
- Constipation
- Muscle cramps
- Abdominal distention

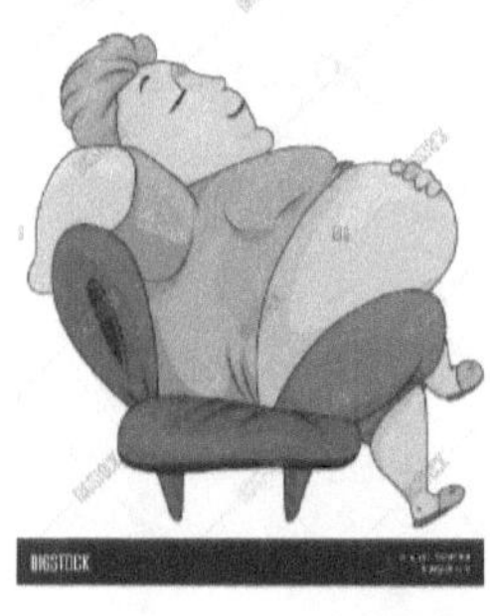

The shortness of breath and muscle cramps may limit exercise and, of course, the abdominal distention will increase clothing size.

Clearly, this is not a good combination for aiding weight loss and feeling better about yourself.

Hypokalaemia needs to be addressed through the replacement of diuretics by another potassium sparing diuretic. However, it always makes good sense to check, on a regular basis, whether diuretics are still needed.

 Reducing salt will help lessen the fluid load and actually drinking more fluid can strangely, help reduce fluid retention.

The underlying reasons why laxatives are required need to be explored since laxatives can, in the long term, cause constipation!

They do this by expelling potassium and magnesium in greater amounts than would normally be expelled.

Both magnesium and potassium are required for the smooth working of the bowel and when they are in short supply abdominal distension and discomfort can occur.

Meanwhile an increase in foods containing potassium should address the abdominal distension.

Foods rich in potassium include

- Bananas
- Plums
- oranges
- Meat
- potatoes
- Tomatoes

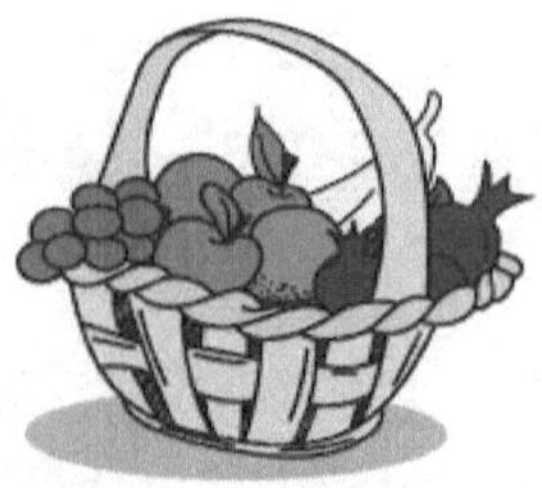

The potassium in many fruits can help any abdominal distention caused by potassium loss through the use of diuretics\laxatives.

Medication for neuropathic pain

Most medication for neuropathic pain such as that prescribed for those with MS has a reputation for piling on the pounds. The reasons for this have been attributed to their ability to increase appetite; they also have a tendency to cause oedema.

Pregabalin is also used for treating epilepsy, shingles pain, diabetic neuropathy and anxiety. This means that, as a whole, these types of medications, which are prescribed widely, are contributing to obesity.

Alternative forms of analgesia will be produced at the end of this book.

Pregabalin works in a number of different ways

- It reduces the electrical activity which causes seizures in those with epilepsy.
- With nerve pain it blocks pain by interfering with the pain messages travelling from the brain to the spine.
- Pregabalin addresses anxiety by preventing your brain from releasing the chemicals that make you feel anxious.

Magnesium, a mineral which is involved in over 700 enzymatic actions in the body, is able to address all the above and may be used to replace Pregabalin and without the associated weight gain.

Antibiotics

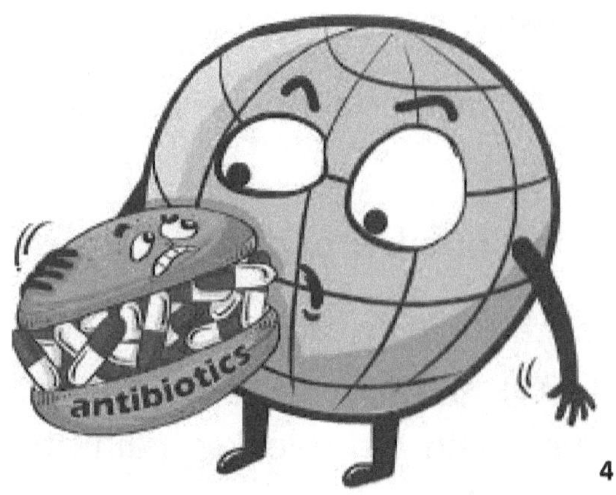

I've taken too many unnecessary antibiotics.

One of the unwanted side effects of antibiotics which tends not to reach the leaflets enclosed with the medication is that can produce significant weight gain.

---

[4] http://www.chinadaily.com.cn/opinion/2016-11/17/content_27401092.htm

Gut bacteria have numerous functions in your body and can play a role in obesity. Studies have shown that exposure to antibiotics in early life may have long term consequences for a child's metabolism.

Mice given antibiotics for the first four weeks of life grew up to be 25% heavier. They also had 60% more body fat than the controls.

Earlier research also showed that mice fed antibiotics – in doses similar to those given to children for throat or ear infections had significant increases in body fat despite their diets remaining unchanged.

There is an association between the composition of the intestinal microbiota and obesity. This has been demonstrated by studies showing differences in microbiota composition between obese and lean humans.

Obesity is associated with an increase of the phylum Firmucutes and a decrease in Bacteroidetes which are partly attributable to diet.

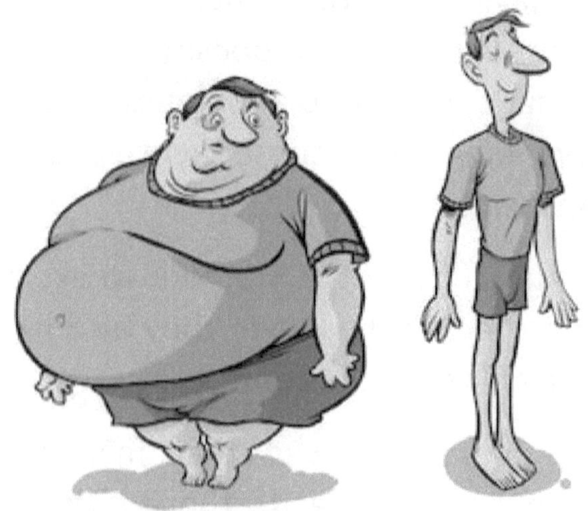

shutterstock.com • 133006715

Left: microbiota of increased Firmucute. Right: microbiota of increased Bacteroidetes

When a low energy diet is taken then there is a shift in gut microbiota with a decrease in Firmucutes.

It has been found that this is similar to the gut bacteria found in a lean person.

When calorie intake is increased then Firmucutes multiplies reflecting the microbiota of obese people.

The judicious use of antibiotics is of paramount importance. Antibiotics do not work on many infectious agents such as viruses and unwise prescribing can lead to antibiotic resistance as well as obesity.

Alternative remedies for common ailments need to be explored. Further, we also need to look at how we can harness our own defences in order to avoid the overuse of antibiotics. Rest, moderate exercise and nutritionally sound meals help our immune systems to function as they should.

Attention should be paid to vitamin D3 and zinc intake in the colder months since they are vital nutrients in fighting infection.   Further, adequate levels of vitamin D3 have been found to be associated with modest reductions in weight.

Case Notes

Joanne was diagnosed with asthma as a child after suffering repeated strep throats and chest infections which required the prescribing of antibiotics.

Joanne was still an active child though but as she grew older, she noticed that, after a course of antibiotics, she put on quite marked amounts of weight which she was unable to shift afterwards. This was in spite of the fact that her appetite had not changed or her calorie intake increased. She still led an active life but she was unable to lose the weight that she had gained even on a very low calorie diet. She had been advised against this because of the danger of loss of muscle mass.

Joanne did not lose weight on this very low calorie diet either and she admitted to feeling desperate.

It was felt that the antibiotics had disrupted her gut bacteria. She was encouraged to eat a wide range of foods including high fibre foods and fermented foods which would help to increase the diversity of gut bacteria.

Joanne is beginning to lose weight without changing her calorie intake.

Cysteine isn't a medication but..........

Cysteine is an amazing amino acid. It is one of the few amino acids which contains sulfur and this allows it bond and maintain the structure of proteins in the body.   Cysteine is also a component of the antioxidant glutathione. It helps maintain strong healthy hair, and blooming skin.

So far so good!

Recent studies have linked cysteine with obesity. Population studies consistently show a positive associate of plasma cysteine with fat mass.

This association appears to be independent of other lifestyle and dietary considerations. It is thought that increased cysteine availability may increase body fat.

Foods high in cysteine are

- Meat, eggs and dairy
- Red peppers, garlic, onions, broccoli, Brussels sprouts, oats, wheat germ, sprouted lentil.

In fact, many of the foods we are encouraged to eat to keep the BMI down!

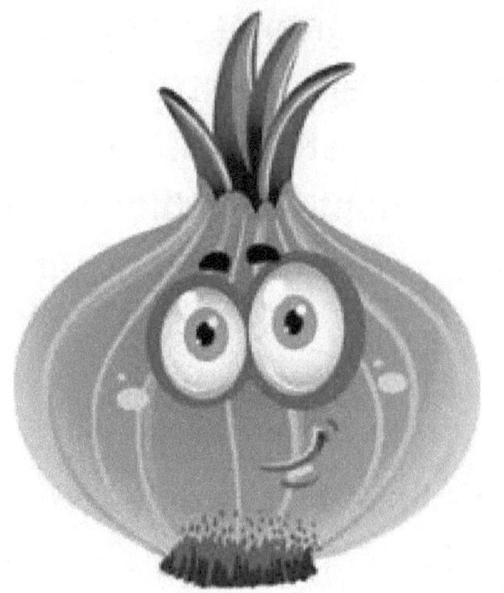

Onions are associated with obesity as they contain cysteine

5

Why calories from sugar increase weight more than calories from other sources.

All cells in your body need glucose for energy. However, it cannot go into your cells directly to fuel them. Once a meal has been taken, blood sugar levels will rise. This will prompt beta cells

---

[5] Clipartpanda.com

in the pancreas to release insulin into your blood stream. This directs muscles and fat cells to take in glucose. The muscles will use glucose for immediate use –some is stored as glycogen for later use. The fat cells will store any glucose – again as glycogen -which is not required immediately.

When glycogen is used up, the muscle protein is broken down into amino acids. The liver can use amino acids to create glucose through a process called glucogenesis. However, this is not as efficient as using glycogen and requires more energy to do so.

Fat stores can be used for energy and form ketones in the process of doing so. The simplest such compound is acetone and this gives the 'pear drop' type odour from someone's breath when they are breaking down fat to use as energy.

It can be seen that if the blood sugar levels are maintained so that they don't spike then there is less likelihood that weight will be gained. This is the science behind the Atkins diet where carbohydrate intake is kept very low and the nutrients are taken from fat and protein sources. The Atkins diet is not about calorie counting. It works purely because it prevents the insulin spikes which start the process of storing energy as fat.

However, there has to be a word of caution here. Many of the vegetable oil types of fat are pro-inflammatory and can, in themselves, cause obesity. While old fashioned lard, butter and dripping are out of favour, they are actually healthy types of fat and provide many health benefits which vegetable oils don't. They are, for example, unlikely to produce free radicals. They are stable when used in cooking.

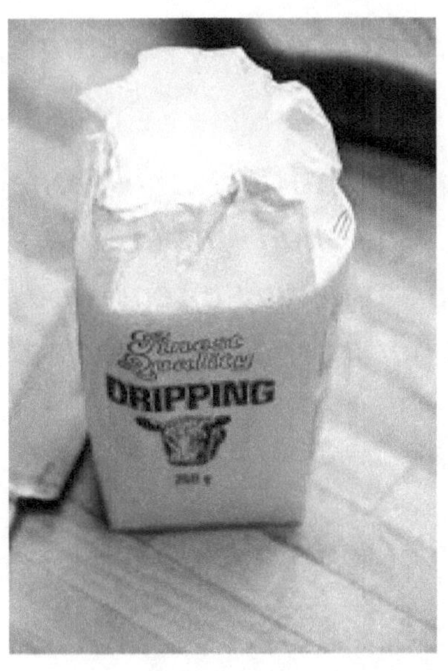

Beef dripping is a stable saturated fat which helps lower cholesterol levels, promotes a healthy skin and does not cause inflammation.

Case notes

Sarah had a diet high in sugary foods and pro-inflammatory oils, the latter of which she thought was healthy. She was about three stone overweight, lacked energy and had joint pain. Her skin was dull and looked dry.

Sarah was encouraged to try an alternative way of eating by reducing the amount of simple carbohydrates and substituting saturated fats like lard, dripping and butter for the vegetable oils and margarine.

Three months later, Sarah had lost one stone and looked healthier. She had much more energy and preferred her new way of eating as it was tastier. She does not intend to go back to her old way of eating.

Other sources of help in weight reduction

Choline - a vital nutrient in weight reduction

Weight reduction is part of the fight in reducing the impact of lymphoedema. It is also a hard fight since when we reduce calories and body mass decreases, the synthesis of the hunger inhibiting hormone, leptin, is also reduced. As a result, hunger pangs increase and it is not long before the diet is abandoned without achieving its aims.

How then can we lose weight without damaging muscle mass and further, making sure that this is undertaken without too much effort on our part. Food is meant to be enjoyed and there is little enjoyment in it when every calorie is being counted on a day to day basis.

A recently discovered nutritional substance which is present in some foods has been found to be the dieter's best friend. Its name is choline and some choline is made in the body but most has to be provided in the food that we eat. Unfortunately, most people are deficient in this vitamin like substance.

What does choline do to help weight loss? Well, choline has been found to help the body use fat as a fuel and further, choline helps to remove excess fat from the blood. When fat is used as a fuel then hunger will not occur.

Studies[6] on the effect of choline supplementation on rapid weight loss and biochemical variables among female taekwondo and judo athletes have born this out. For a number of reasons, it is necessary for athletes to lose weight before important matches. This is undertaken using a number of nutritional substances of which one is choline. Dramatic weight loss without the loss of muscle mass has been observed in those taking choline supplementation.

The athletes took 2g of choline daily - divided into two 1g doses - for one week. The results indicated a 10.23% change in loss of body fat. The results support the hypothesis that choline

---

[6] https://www.ncbi.nlm.nih.gov/pmc/articles/PMC4096089/#b4-jhk-40-77

could be used to lose weight rapidly without detriment to other body systems.

Good sources of choline are eggs and liver. Two eggs provide about half of the choline requirements for the day.

A Recommended Daily Allowance has not been established for choline since it is a fairly newly discovered substance. However, an Adequate Intake has been established and this is:

- 425mg for women
- 550mg for men

Some individuals will require less than this and others more. There are a number of groups of people who are likely to require more and, as such be at risk of being deficient in choline. These groups are:

- Anyone with a poor diet or malabsorption problems
- Pregnant mothers
- Nursing mothers
- The elderly
- Vegetarians and vegans

The best sources of choline are foods which are now advised as those that may increase cholesterol levels. As such they are avoided. In addition, the best source of choline – beef liver - has fallen out of popularity. When we take eggs and liver out of the diet then it can be seen that achieving the adequate intake of choline is not easy.

Foods containing choline

- One large egg: 120mg
- Beef liver: one slice contains 280mg
- Salmon: 4 ounces contains 65mg
- Cod: 85gms contains 250mg
- Cauliflower: 120ml contains 25mg
- Broccoli: 120ml contains 24mg
- Brussels sprouts: one cup cooked 65mg
- Soybean oil: one tablespoon contains 47mg
- Peanut butter: one tablespoon 10mg

It can be see that it is considerably harder to obtain adequate intakes of choline in a plant based diet than it is for those who include meat in their meals.

There should be no fear in eating eggs. One of Choline's functions is to lower cholesterol levels and as eggs contain superb amounts of choline then the hype that they can contribute to heart disease and stroke is unfounded. Choline can also lower blood pressure.

It makes sense to increase levels of choline in the diet. This is not an overly difficult thing to achieve. For example, stirring a couple of egg yolks into mashed potato before topping a shepherd's pie or making proper Crème Anglaise with egg yolks goes well towards the Adequate Intake of choline. Making a shepherd's pie with minced liver is also a tried and tested recipe in our household. I make this with lamb's liver as the flavour is more delicate than that of beef liver. However, it depends on individual taste. Liver is such a good all round food that it is eaten twice weekly in our house.

If cooking is not your forte, then supplements are useful and easily obtainable online and in health food stores. It is recommended that no more than 600mg is taken daily but be guided by the instructions on the pack.

Amino acids are a major source of help in the fight in reducing weight. Our weight – whether gained or lost – is mainly down to the amino acids and their ability to stimulate the body to produce enough fat burning hormones.

The growth hormone somatotropin is a major player in this field. We produce this hormone while we sleep so already you can see that poor sleep quality is likely to lead to weight gain.

Somatotropin stimulates protein synthesis and boosts fat burning. It requires certain amino acids in order to do this and these amino acids must be taken at night on an empty stomach.

These amino acids are

- Methionine
- Arginine
- Glutamine

As well as the above amino acids, vitamin B6, B12 and zinc are required.

Methionine is found in sulphurous foods such as egg yolk, green leafy vegetables, garlic and onions.

Arginine is found in chicken, turkey, pork loin, soybeans, peanuts and dairy.

See glutamine sources below.

Carnitine is a compound which helps transport long chain fatty acids into the mitochondria so that they can be burned to produce energy. Without carnitine this would not happen although medium and short chain fatty acids can pass without this transport molecule.

It is found in liver. This is not surprising since carnitine is synthesised in the liver. Its precursor is made in the kidneys and requires two essential amino acids, lysine and methionine.

As carnitine transports fatty acids into the metabolic furnace so quickly, the body is more likely to burn fat than store it.

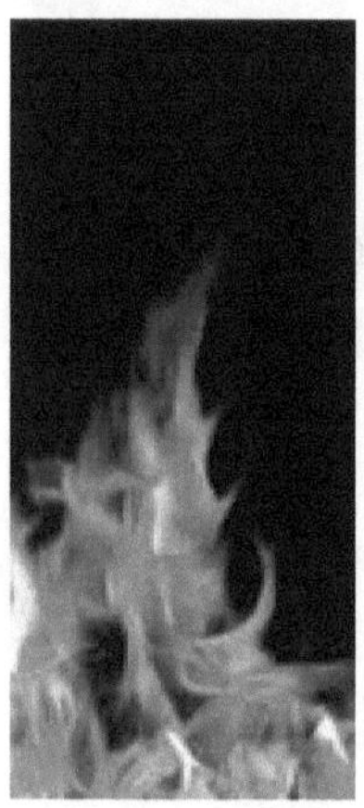

Carnitine transports fatty acids into mitochondria quickly so that the body is more likely to burn fat than store it.

Studies by scientists from Switzerland and the USA have proved that carnitine can increase the mobilisation of fatty acids from fat cells and well as increase the burning of those fatty acids in the cells.

Carnitine's benefits for weight loss do not end there. Supplementation of carnitine during a calorie reduced diet not only increases fat loss but provides a simultaneous increase in muscle mass.

Glutamine counteracts fat storage. This amino acid can be converted to glucose in the kidneys and doesn't affect glucagon. As glutamine counteracts fat storage it can have comparable results with medications such as Alli, a weight loss aid, which works to prevent fat from being absorbed.

Glucagon is a hormone which is produced in the pancreas. It helps to raise the concentration of glucose and fatty acids in the bloodstream.

Glutamine doesn't affect insulin levels either. Therefore, it can contribute to the energy supply. However, it is able to do this without affecting insulin levels and insulin induced fat storage.

In conclusion, glutamine counteracts the storage of dietary fats and therefore helps to regulate weight.

Studies have even shown that when glutamine is administered in a high fat diet it still resulted in a loss of body fat. It can also reduce cravings for sugar and alcohol.

Glutamine is stored in muscles and is a conditional amino acid. This means that the body can make it but, at times of stress or illness or injury, it may need supplementing.

Glutamine powder is easily available in health food stores or online. It is tasteless and can be sprinkled over food. Up to 15g daily can be taken in three divided doses.

Good sources of glutamine are:

- Seafood
- Meat
- Milk
- Eggs
- Protein powders (whey)
- Cabbage
- Beans

Phenylalanine as an appetite suppressant

Phenylalanine is an essential amino acid which means that we have to get it from external sources. It works as an appetite suppressant and effects this by assisting the release of a hormone called cholecystokinin. This tells the brain to feel full when you have eaten.

As food hits the stomach food enters the stomach, this hormone directs digestion to slow down. Appetite decreases. This generally occurs after 20 minutes. This explains why people who eat more slowly are likely to be thinner than those who eat more quickly. This amino acid is found in a number of foods including:

- Brown rice
- Bananas
- Eggs
- Fish
- Peanuts
- Sesame seeds
- Nuts especially almonds

The downside is, that in order to get an effective amount you would need to eat a lot of foods containing phenylalanine. However, in matters of weight loss where other methods haven't worked then phenylalanine supplementation may be considered.

Phenylalanine has a number of other benefits too. It is very successful at treating severe pain. A reduction in pain can help reduced elevated cortisol levels that are a result of the stress that pain carries with it; cortisol, as we have already seen is a major player in weight gain.

By now you have probably realised that food cravings do not start in your stomach. Hunger starts in your brain and appetite is controlled by a part of the brain known as the hypothalamus.

The hypothalamus receives many messages from hormones which are secreted from various parts of the body such as the pancreas, fat cells and intestines. This all helps to regulate and control hunger.

There are many other factors which influence hunger and these include:

- rise in blood sugar and insulin
- stress
- the palatability of food
- rise in the hunger hormone, leptin
- conditioned responses
- variety of food on offer – the greater the variety of food the more we are likely to eat
- boredom
- the amount and type of amino acids in the diet
- sunlight

Stress and weight gain

In our fast moving lives of the 21st century, one of the negative effects of this is unhealthy weight gain. Three hormones are involved in this process:

- Epinephrine
- Norepinephrine
- Cortisol

The first two hormones are released when under stress and help release cortisol. Cortisol provides energy in readiness for the fight or flight response. stimulates the release of insulin and fat and carbohydrate metabolism. If the stressful event continues then this pattern of eating high fat and high carbohydrate food occurs. Eating foods which overall, are not healthy, is not a sign of greed or lack of self-control, it is a very real issue caused by high levels of cortisol circulating in the system.

Stress has also been found to inhibit serotonin – a chemical messenger which promotes feelings of calm. Eating carbohydrates promotes the synthesis of serotonin which is why - when people are feeling stressed - they crave sweet foods.

Animal research has further supported the link between stress and obesity. Rats were given the rodent version of cortisol. This induced a state associated with chronic stress. When concentrations of cortisol rose, the rats ate more lard and drank more sugar water. As a result, their abdominal girth increased. These type of foods seem to calm the body's response to stress. Further, they may be eaten in response to perceived threats where the fight or flight response may be instigated that requires a ready source of energy.

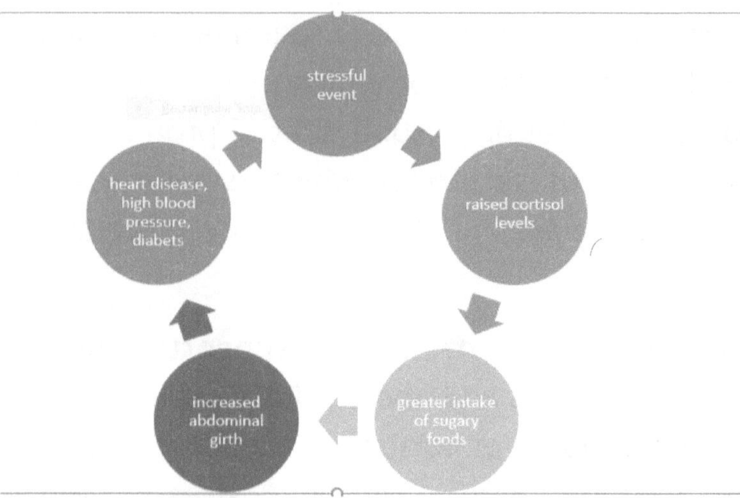

The downward cycle of stress.

Cortisol also encourages the formation of fat cells. These 'stress' associated fat cells will be deposited on the abdomen rather than the thighs. This abdominal fat is associated with heart disease, high blood pressure and diabetes.

There are a number of ways that cortisol levels can be reduced. These are:

- Take DHEA
- Melatonin
- B vitamins
- Magnesium

- L-theanine

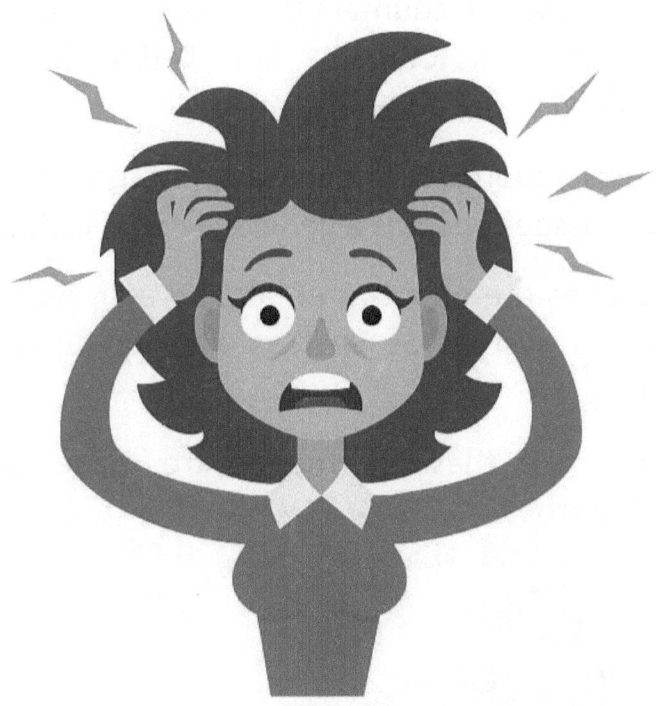

Stress promotes the release of cortisol which helps to lay down fat.

Dehydroepiandsterone (DHEA) is an adrenal hormone which counters the effect of cortisol in many tissues. Cortisol, like DHEA, is also produced in the adrenal glands.

Cortisol suppresses the immune system, breaks down tissues and has a general catabolic effect.

DHEA has the opposite effect and activates the immune system as well as helping build up tissues.

Both of these hormones are made from cholesterol.

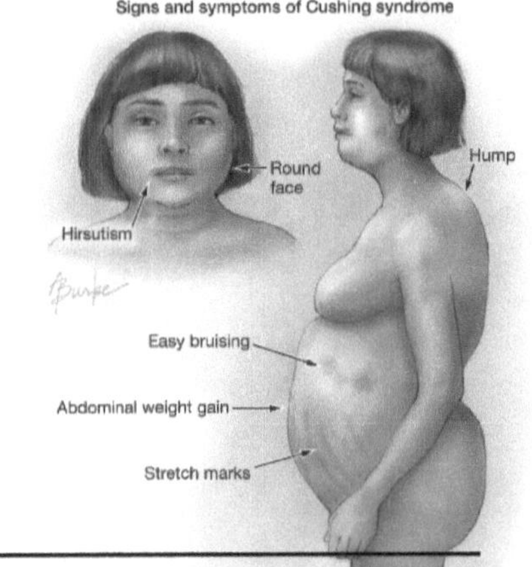

[7]

Too much cortisol lays down fat in this distribution

---

[7] https://jamanetwork.com/journals/jama/fullarticle/1104780

Both of these hormones are essential for life. Too much cortisol is associated with Cushing's Syndrome which is associated with high blood sugar levels, weight gain, fragile skin, rosy, healthy looking cheeks, weakening bones and weight gain around the abdomen.

Too little cortisol results in Addison's disease and is due to adrenal gland damage. In this scenario there will be unintentional weight loss.

In matters of L-theanine, studies[8] have shown that intake of this amino acid resulted in a reduction in the heart rate and salivary immunoglobulin A (IgA) response which is an immune system antibody. It was found that the control group who were not given L-theanine had much lower levels of IgA.

---

[8] https://www.ncbi.nlm.nih.gov/pubmed/16930802

This antibody helps keep parts of the body which are lined with mucous cells such as the respiratory tract and bowel, healthy. It follows that stress can lower the body's resistance to disease.

Clearly, stress can induce obesity so is there anything that can help reduce stress levels and the ongoing effects of stress?

Magnesium increases the production of GABA which helps to encourage relaxation as well as sleep. Magnesium also helps to regulate the body's stress response.

One small trial of 43 elderly people in Tehran looked at the effect of 500mg of magnesium on the quality of sleep. Those who received the supplement of magnesium fell asleep quicker and spent more of their time in bed but their total sleep time was not necessarily longer.

GABA can be taken as a supplement before bedtime. 500mg should be sufficient although some people take twice this much. Be guided by the instructions that come with it.

Magnesium can be taken at a dose of 500mg before bed. It can cause diarrhoea so be guided by this. You may need to start off with a smaller dose and work your way up until you find the correct dose for you.

L-theanine is normally taken at 200mg twice a day although this can be raised to four times a day if this lower does is not effective. There are very few sources of L-theanine but it can be found in green and black tea which will explain why a cup of tea is normally offered to someone at times of stressful situations.

As L-theanine can reduce the heart rate, then anyone with a naturally slow heart rate should not consider taking L-theanine until they have discussed this with someone who is medically qualified.

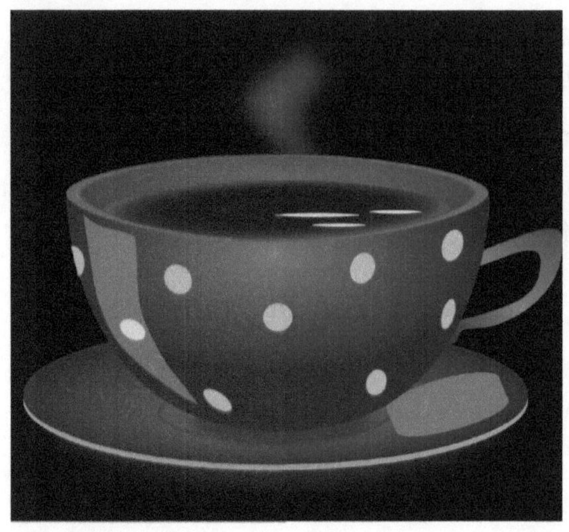

In relation to vitamin B, one table can be taken in the morning as opposed to night time. Vitamin B releases energy which is not what we want when we are trying to sleep.

 Melatonin can be taken at doses of 3mg daily before bedtime. However, it is recommended that the individual combine gentle exercise with daylight hours. This practise should increase the synthesis of melatonin during the darker hours.

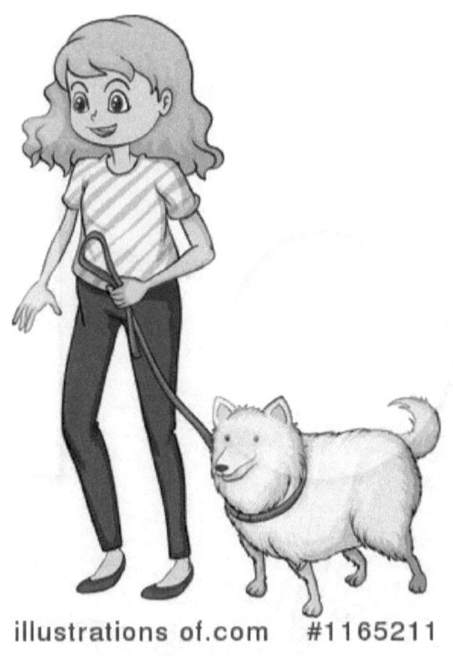

Gently exercise in daylight helps relieve stress.

Part of coping with stress is having the forethought to plan ahead for any unforeseen eventualities which may occur. This may involve keeping a rainy day fund for unexpected occurrences; keeping important dates and, telephone numbers, for example, in appropriate places so that they are to hand, also helps to alleviate stress. It hardly goes without saying that those who are disorganised are also chronically stressed. Difficult times will happen to all of us but we can lessen the impact that they are likely to have on us with a little forethought.

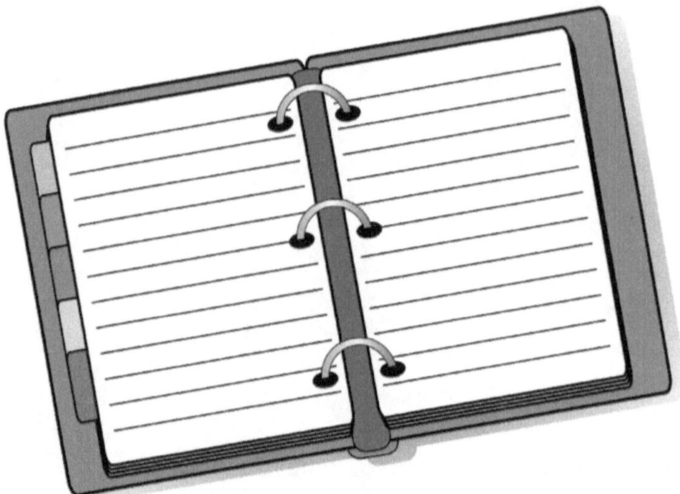

Keeping important dates in a planner and making sure that you make time for yourself are necessary to reduce the impact of stress.

Sunlight

Why does sunlight have the potential to reduce body weight?

Firstly, studies have found that the sun's blue light wavelengths can penetrate our skin. Blue light is the light that we can see with our eye. If blue light reaches the fat cells just beneath our skin, the lipid droplets reduce in size and are released from the cell. This may account for the loss of weight that many people encounter in the summer months.

Melatonin, the hormone responsible for the sleep wake cycle has been found to speed up the production of fat burning. Of course, melatonin production decreases in the presence of light, you might argue. However, intense light – such as that found in sunlight – while completely eliminating melatonin in the body, helps increase its production at night. Following on from this, we can deduce that anything which interferes with the production of melatonin, can potentially cause weight gain.

Anyone, therefore, who works in an office environment, under yellow lights, is potentially increasing their risk of gaining unwanted weight.

There are many lamps designed for those with seasonal affective disorder (SAD). They give out the blue ultra violet light which we require to completely eliminate melatonin from the body during the day. The regulation of the sleep wake cycle is set properly by these lamps.

If obesity is caused by the lack of blue light this type of lamp should treat the cause adequately.

Normally, it is advised that individuals sit in front of the SAD boxes for a minimum of thirty minutes so that the light enters the eye. It is possible to carry on working as this is happening.

The minimum lux required is 2,000 lux which is four times brighter than office lights, on average.

Blue light is emitted from the screens of computers, electronic notebooks, smartphones and other digital devices.   However, this is nowhere near the amount that is emitted by the sun. Nevertheless, the amounts of light are significant enough to to prevent sleep, if people have been looking at screens before they go to bed.

Case history

Peter was a very active person. He was not overly slim but, in the winter, he put on about two stone in weight. He was tired, irritable and kept complaining that it was too dark for him to be motivated to do anything. He constantly raided the fridge. Shortly after the shortest day, he began to improve slowly, taking a more active interest in life and eating less.
Peter was encouraged to get out into daylight as early in the morning as he could. He bought a SAD box and spent about an hour in front of it

when he was at work. He did become less irritable and found that he did not eat as much. He only gained about half a stone over the winter period instead of the two stone that had been the norm. This was much more acceptable to him and his wife.

Artificial Sweeteners

Artificial sweeteners are widely used as replacements for sugar. Some studies have shown that they can negatively affect gut bacteria. Other studies do not have the same finding. So are they safe or not and do they contribute to weight gain?

Studies have shown that the artificial sweetener aspartame reduced weight gain but it also increased blood sugar and impaired insulin response. However, these studies were conducted on animals and far larger doses were used than humans would be likely to ingest on a daily basis. Further, sweeteners have passed rigorous safety tests before being allowed for sale.

When ingested sweeteners are broken down into components that the body can use to build up materials it does want. In this respect, they behave like any other food that we take in. Food is broken down in digestion, waste is eliminated and the useful bits are used to make whatever material is required   by the body at the time.

Aspartame, for example, is broken down into two amino acids – aspartic acid and phenylalanine. A third substance – a non- amino acid, methanol, is also produced.

Phenylalanine has been found to be a natural painkiller and appetite suppressant, so clearly aspartame is useful once it is broken down in the body.

Aspartic acid can increase the release of a hormone in the brain that will result eventually in testosterone production. Studies do not show that it has any effect on weight gain.

Methanol is the simplest alcohol and is found occurring in small quantities in the body. Many people will not entertain sweeteners because of this side effect. However, the amount of methanol that is produced from the breakdown of is miniscule compared to the amount that is produced in the process of breaking down foodstuffs consumed on a day to day basis.

Humans are programmed to like sweet things. It is a survival strategy in case we require large amounts of energy to fuel the flight or fight response. Of course, we do not need large amounts of readily available energy on a day to day level anymore. However, we still have stressors which challenge us and induce the release of cortisol and the subsequent need for energy.

The nature of our stressors appear to have changed. We no longer have to watch out for marauding carnivores or enemies likely to carry off wives and children. Most of our stressors are sedentary ones; how do we pay the mortgage? Will our children do well at school?

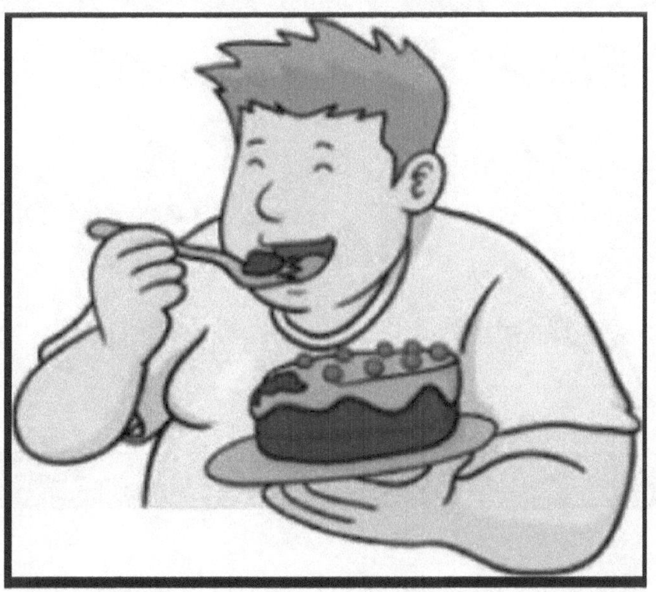

[9] **Human beings are programmed to like sweet things.**

---

[9] https://www.kisspng.com/png-birthday-cake-chocolate-cake-fast-food-clip-art-re-1406881/preview.html

These stressors do not use the energy up in physical activity as would have once occurred. Nevertheless, we still demand sweet things but do not use the calories up in the fight or flight response.

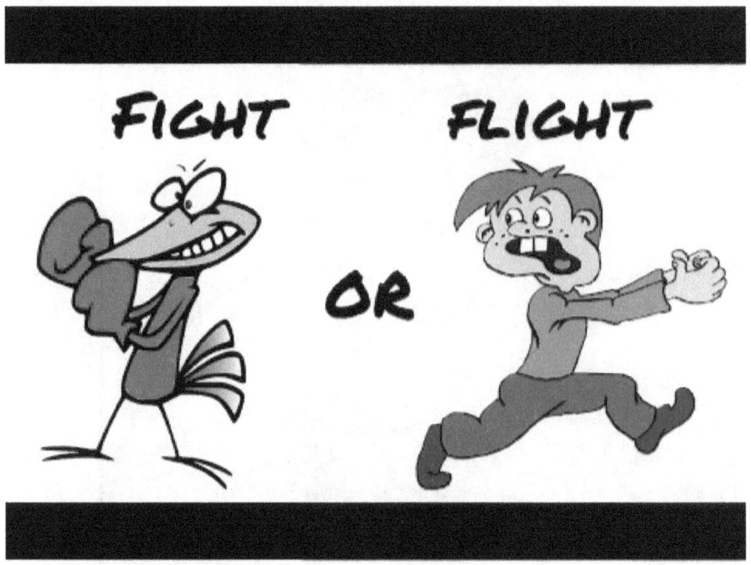

10 **The fight or flight response, in response to perceived threat uses energy.**

If you have a sweet tooth and cannot resist sweet things regardless of whether you need

---

10 https://www.youtube.com/watch?v=mtRrxNTnyh8

the energy or not, then I cannot see a problem in using proprietary sweeteners to sweeten food you would normally sweeten with sugar. Diabetics do this, after all. The only caveat is that some artificial sweeteners do contain calories even if they contain less than sugar, like for like.

However, now is probably a good time to try out some recipes that provide energy but do not result in the harmful spikes of blood sugar that encourage the storage of fat in fat cells

Here is an example, below.

<u>Recipe for a sugarless pudding.</u>

A cupful of mashed cooked carrots

2-3 tablespoons of desiccated coconut

A grated apple

A cupful of dried fruit soaked in cold tea

A tsp of mixed spice

Artificial sweetener to taste

 2-3 eggs

 Self-raising flour or ground almonds or a combination of both – enough to produce a pudding consistency.

50g of butter (but this can be left out and does not detract from the taste or texture).

Method

Mix all together, place in a pudding basin and steam for two hours. Serve with a little yogurt.

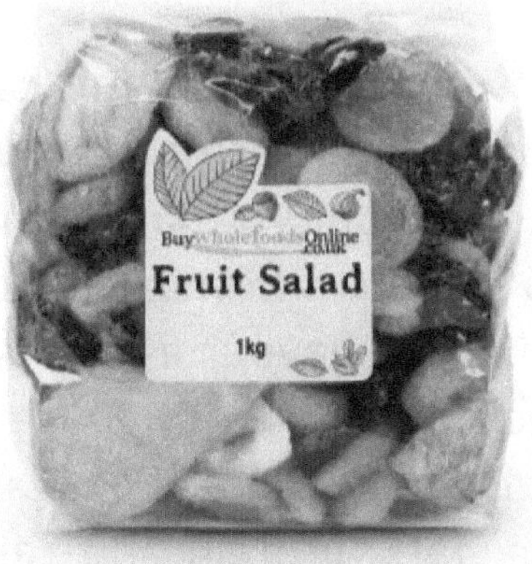

Dried fruit provides fibre as well as sweetness.

The apple, carrot and dried fruit provide most of the sweetness. This is one of our favourite puddings as it is also very healthy on a number of levels. It is full of antioxidants.

This pudding mix can also be baked in a lined loaf tin at 180C for 40 minutes depending on how much flour you have used and how 'dry' the cake mix is. As is usual, test it with the blade of a knife to see if the mixture has cooked. You may need to cover the top of the cake and cover with foil if it is in danger of burning.

I use a lot of vegetables in my cakes. Most people will have tried carrot cake or chocolate beetroot cake but did you know that adding a tin of tomato soup to a fruit cake endows it with moisture and a rich flavour as well as loading it with lycopene? It's all good, dense nutrition; a little goes a long way and it is a meal in itself. It contains fibre, fats, protein and carbohydrates as well as numerous antioxidants and trace minerals, macronutrients and vitamins. A slice is not a quick snack because we don't have time for a meal. It **is** the complete meal in all its glory.

Sometimes I make extra and steam it as a pudding; it tastes wonderful however you cook it.

Here is a recipe you may like to try.

Tomato soup cake

Ingredients

Two cups of flour
Two cups of dried fruit (soaked in cold tea)
One cup of sugar
100g of butter or less
Three eggs
Two teaspoons of mixed spice
One teaspoon of bicarbonate of soda
One tin of tomato soup (400g)
Walnuts as desired (keep some back for the top
of the cake but put the rest, ground up, into the
cake mix.
Vanilla essence
Cream cheese
Few drops of liquid sweetener

Method

Place all the ingredients into a bowl **apart from
the vanilla essence, liquid sweetener and
cream cheese.** Mix well.

Place into a lined container and bake for about
45 minutes at 180C. The cake is ready when a
skewer is inserted and comes out clean.

Decorate the top with a little cream cheese mixed with vanilla essence and a few drops of liquid sweetener. Decorate with walnuts, as desired.

Adenosine

Not many people have heard of adenosine never mind know what it does. Adenosine is a regulatory molecule in metabolic processes. Therefore, it is vital for health.

In the brain, adenosine is a neurotransmitter (brain chemical) that has an inhibitory action. It promotes sleep. Levels of adenosine rise throughout the day in response to exercise. At the end of the day provided adenosine levels are high enough then arousal is suppressed and sleep promoted.

Adenosine has many other actions including energy metabolism and expenditure.

The more physical exercise that you do the more the more adenosine is produced. Adenosine helps muscles to adapt to exercise thus helping to prevent trauma. In addition, adenosine is also released in response to:

- Trauma of any kind
- Oxidative stress — where it helps to protect the brain
- Metabolic distress

Adenosine is found in all organs in the body where it has a diversity of functions including:

Kidneys – decreased blood flow and decreased production of rennin from the kidney

Lungs – constriction of airways

Liver – constriction of blood vessels and increased breakdown of glycogen to form glucose

Heart – decreased heart rate and has antiplatelet action and increased diameter of blood vessels in peripheral organs

Adenosine's numerous functions include:

- Relaxing vascular smooth muscle
- Regulating T cell proliferation and cytokine production - cytokines are small proteins that are secreted by cells of the immune system and have an effect on other cells.
- Relieving nerve pain including shingles
- **Inhibiting lipolysis**

Inhibiting lipolysis is the one that we are interested in. Lipolysis is the breakdown of fat. Fats are broken down in our body by enzymes and water. Fat is actually stored energy and found in adipose tissue stores. Fat has many uses including cushioning our bodies from trauma. Excess calories – over and above our needs – are stored as triglycerides and broken down when we need the energy that is stored there. This energy is useful in times of illness when appetite is lost. The stored fat is broken down into fatty acids and glycerol. Adenosine is used in the composition of adenosine triphosphate, also known as ATP.

ATP provides energy which is required to fuel many of the processes in living cells. For example, you cannot contract muscles without it or initiate nerve impulses.

The importance of ATP is demonstrated by its description of

The molecular unit of currency of intracellular energy transfer

Now ATP is synthesised from fatty acids and protein from lean meats - chicken and turkey, for example, and also from fatty fish and nuts. However, as adenosine inhibits lipolysis, eating these foods – including chicken and turkey – have to potential to increase weight gain or the breakdown of fat for fuel. This may take some time to get your head around. We are so used to hearing that turkey and chicken are ideal foods for weight loss and in some respects – within a calorie controlled diet - they may be. However, we cannot look at any food in the light of how many calories a portion contains. Any food has numerous nutritional substances contained within it and each of those will interact with an individual's genetic makeup and impact on many aspects of overall health.

As adenosine containing foods are essential for energy transfer then we should not seek to limit them from our diet. However, we need to be aware that too many may – in genetically susceptible people – carry the risk for unwanted weight gain which is difficult to lose. Reducing the amount of foods containing adenosine during calorie restriction would aid the breakdown of stored fat.

The actions of adenosine are antagonised by theophylline. The main source of theophylline is cocoa bean. Therefore, it is quite possible to lose weight eating very dark chocolate with a high cocoa composition of 85% or over. Drinking cocoa or eating dark chocolate, high in cocoa solids, helps the breakdown of fat. In addition, tea also contains modest amounts of theophylline.

Theophylline is a Methylxanthines. Methylxanthines have a role as antagonists of A_1 and A_2 adenosine receptors. Caffeine and theobromine are the most abundant naturally occurring of Methylxanthines.

Theobromine – also found in cocoa – improves your circulation and respiratory system. It increases the activity of a cell called cyclic adenosine monophosphate (cAMP). This messenger molecule activates an enzyme which reduces inflammation.

Given the impact of cocoa as a super food, why dark chocolate with very high amounts of cocoa solids, is often limited - in weight loss diets – to a couple of squares is beyond me. It can be eaten in greater quantities and more often than is normally advised.

On a personal level, I have found that when my intake of dark chocolate goes up replacing desserts – although the calories or more or less equal – I always lose significant amounts of weight during that period.

Final Thoughts

When I considered writing a book on weight, I noticed how many books were written on numerous diets which often left the dieter feeling deprived and further, did nothing to address the issue about weight gain; that is, it often has other causes than intake of more calories than is expended which is what is generally mooted.

Research has shown that calories from foods containing the amino acid, methionine has the potential to cause weight gain while those containing amino acids like L-theanine, GABA and glutamine all have the potential to cause weight loss. Thus, it can be seen that not all calories are the same.

 It is these issues which I wished to address in this book.

As a lecturer and medical nutritionist, I am also aware that, until individuals have some idea why and how appetite and weight gain occur, then they are unlikely to be able to understand and engage wholeheartedly with addressing the issues – if they still feel that they need to be addressed.

I make no apology for not including lists of recipes for dieters. There are plenty of books out there for those who want a book on low calorie meals. Weight loss is not about deprivation. Food is meant to be enjoyed and not every obese person is unhealthy. Conversely, not every slim person is healthy, either.

Our perceptions of ourselves are influenced by prevailing fashion and our body shape may be the desired shape in one decade but not so in the next.

As I believe I have demonstrated, any body shape and feature can be an asset. We should not be slaves to popular fashion. We can be our own person and be confident in that. Confidence, is after all the best fashion item we can wear – that and a smile.

My hope is that you can take something from
this book which will change your life for the
better.

Amino acids, antioxidant, anti-inflammatory and pain relieving properties which don't cause weight gain.

Amino acids are the building blocks of protein and, as such are found in all animal foods Peas, beans and other legumes are rich sources of animal protein.

Amino acids can be non–essential, that is they can be made in the body, or essential which means they must be taken in through diet. Some amino acids are also said to be conditional which means that normally the body can make them but at times of illness or injury, they may need to be ingested or supplemented.

Methionine, cartilage and arthritis.

Professor and Dr Klaus Miehlke was classed as the leading expert on bone diseases in Germany. He has argued that in cases of joint or cartilage disease, it is of the utmost importance that the human body receives the cartilage-forming substances in sufficient quantities. He states that a healthy diet cannot provide this and recommends supplements which contain cartilage-forming substances.

Methionine is one such cartilage forming substance. It is an essential amino acid which means it must be taken in from the diet.

Methionine donates sulphur and joint cartilage requires sulphur for its creation. Tests have shown that cartilage in healthy individuals contains around three times more sulphur than in patients who suffer from arthritis. Patients who have arthritis are advised to supplement with methionine and the B vitamins to optimise the results.

Methionine has particular importance in three main areas

- it stimulates the cartilage cells to create more cartilaginous tissue

- contains anti- inflammatory properties

- has an analgesic effect

Dietary sources of methionine include onions, garlic, eggs, meat, fish, sesame seeds, nuts. Most fruit and vegetables contain little methionine although sulphur containing compounds are found in Brussels sprouts and broccoli.

Arginine helps create new bone therefore it is particularly useful for those with a propensity towards osteoporosis.

Arginine supports the production of collagen which is a protein and is a basic component of connective tissues like cartilage. It also supports the growth of osteoblasts which are cells which form new bone.

When a deficiency of arginine occurs it can cause osteoporosis. Studies have shown that arginine in combination with other amino acids supported the growth of osteoblasts[11] It was therefore recommended that the administration of amino acids belonged to all osteoporosis treatments. Arginine is found in all animal foods, soybeans, peanuts, walnuts and pumpkin seeds.

DL Phenylalanine – this essential amino acid has been well researched and documented and is effective in the control of chronic and acute pain syndromes which include

- lower back pain

- osteoarthritis

---

[11] Ursini, F. & Pipicelli, G. (2009) *Nutritional Supplementation for Osteoarthritis,* Alternative and Complementary Therapies, Volume 15, issue 4, (pp. 173-177)

- joint pain resulting from rheumatoid arthritis

- migraine

- neuralgia

among others

DLPA appears to focus on chronic pain only. It protects the brain own natural endorphins allowing them to continue to act effectively and for longer periods than that of pharmaceutical products.

DLPA has also been found to have strong antidepressant action and is effective in relieving anxiety.

Good sources of phenylalanine are animal foods and beans and nuts. During illness when appetite is lost and phenylalanine levels are also below optimum levels then pain is likely to increase. Phenylalanine supplementation should be considered at this time and is available in powdered form and is obtainable for health food shops or online.

Dosage initial dosage would be 2000mg increasing to no more than 4,500mg by two weeks. It is a good adjunctive therapy but can also be used alone.

Amino acids should always be taken on an empty stomach to maximise absorption. In free form they need no digesting and so can act within minutes – far quicker than prescribed medications unless they are the injectable form.

Glutamine is found in muscles. It is known as brain fuel as it easily passes through the blood brain barrier. Glutamine increases the amount of GABA – another amino acid and neurotransmitter - which inhibits pain. It is the amino acid found in the intestinal gut lining and helps conditions such as Crohn's disease, leaky gut syndrome and irritable bowel syndrome. Thus it helps address gut related pain and any damage caused by NSAID's such as ibuprofen.

The body's two primary pain modulators

The body has its own analgesic system which are the neurotransmitters. The two main ones are derived from amino acids

- Gamma amino butyric acid (GABA)

- Endorphins

It is perhaps no surprise that one of these precursor amino acids is DL phenylalanine. Seymour Ehrenpreis PhD., pharmacology professor at Chicago Medical School demonstrated that this endorphinase[12] allowed the medical school to significantly reduce the amounts of opiate medication administered.

Phenylalanine is also useful in reducing food cravings and can assist in weight loss.

GABA

---

[12] inhibits the breakdown of pain reliving endorphins

GABA is a major inhibitory neurotransmitter and helps calm pain and relieve anxiety. It is also an amino acid in its own right. For a long time GABA was not thought capable of crossing the blood brain barrier but more recently evidence has been found for the presence of a GABA transporter in the blood brain barrier. This demonstrates that GABA can enter or exit the brain.

A lack of inhibition by neurotransmitters – mainly GABA – is responsible for many pain states. Some GABA analogues such as Gabapentin and Pregabalin act by inhibiting ion channels which contributes to their analgesic effects.

While we are on the subject of GABA. It is important to realise that GABA cannot be synthesised with adequate amounts of vitamin B1. Currently, the UK and most of the world are deficient in thiamine. The effects of supplementation with thiamine which can build up over a period of 6 months are nothing short of remarkable. Thiamine in addition to riboflavin – vitamin B2 – also helps in the synthesis of melatonin which is needed for sleep. People report a full night's, refreshing sleep without any hangover effects the following day. Thiamine is a remarkable vitamin which has no upper tolerable limits and has not been found to be contraindicated with any other medication or condition, whatsoever.

Table showing common analgesics, mode of action, dosage and any considerations before administering

.

Nutrient	Mode of Action	Dosage	considerations
Thiamine (vitamin B1)	Diverse and numerous. A deficiency mimics most health conditions. Needed to make GABA – a powerful pain inhibitor	General use: 100mg daily Therapeutic use 300mg daily. When symptoms resolve drop to 100mg Neurodegenerative and intractable chronic disease: 500mg three times daily, rising to 4000mg as necessary until symptoms begin to	Thiamine has been found to have no upper tolerable limit and is therefore safe to use. It is not known to have detrimental effects on any known medications Metformin depletes thiamine

		resolve. Then reduce as necessary.	as does raw fish – sushi and shellfish – a high carb diet, coffee, tea. Should be taken with other B complex as the B vitamins work together synergisti cally
Potassi um	Alleviates pain by increasing the potassium ion channel	Should be taken in food such as bananas and fruit	Should not be suppleme nted unless under medical supervisio

	activity		n. Potassium works within a narrow range and too much or too little can be harmful
capsaicin	Pain receptors become exhausted quickly if an ointment containing capsaicin is used.	Found in peppers which have similar effects when eaten	Can be irritating to the skin in susceptible people
Glutamine and GABA(do not get glutamine	Glutamate increases GABA (as does thiamine). GABA inhibits pain. A lack	See recommendations for thiamine above. Glutamine is found in.	Useful for Crohn's disease, ulcerative colitis, rheumatoid arthritis

mixed up with glutamate, they are entirely different	of which is responsible for many pain states	Clinical trials have used between 5-45g.	and IBS in addition to other pain syndromes. A good all rounder
Curcumin and ginger	Similar to glutamine	As advised on the container	Curcumin is said to help memory. It is anti-inflammatory in nature. Buy curcumin not turmeric as there is very little curcumin in turmeric. Ginger is also stated to

			dampen nausea in addition to having the benefits of curcumin
The amino acid methio nine	Methionine Stimulates cartilage cells to produce more cartilage, it is anti-inflammatory and analgesic. Arginine helps in the synthesis of new bone and cartilage thus preventing the pain caused by the	Methionine is found in sulphur containing foods such as onions, garlic, broccoli. The RDI is 19mg/Kg Arginine is normally taken in therapeutic doses at 2-3g three times	A wide range of applicatio ns but especially conditions such as arthritis. Osteopor osis

	conditions caused by a lack of	daily.	
Vitamin E	Vitamin E has antioxidant activity. It helps protect fatty acids in the brain. It slows down neurodegeneration and the potential for microglia to develop and maintain chronic pain	400 IU's daily	It is a fat soluble vitamin found in wheat germ, nuts and whole wheat products

Vitamin C	Powerful anti - inflammatory and antioxidant	1g daily, increasing with infection, stress and	Very high doses may inhibit thiamine

		injury	
Vitamin A	Neutralises oxidants thereby reducing inflammatory processes	Fat soluble found in full fat dairy. Lots of highly coloured vegetables contain beta carotene which is a precursor to vitamin A. Eat with a little butter for absorption RD1 for adults is 600-800 IU's	Liver is probably the food that contains the most vitamin A so much so that it is not recommended for pregnant women due to risk of foetal malformation.
Magnesium	It is a natural channel blocker. Calcium is one of the	400mg daily Found in a wide range of meat,	People with kidney disease should consult

	most pro-inflammatory substances that there are. So magnesium reduces inflammation. It also reduces substance P and glutamate which transmit pain throughout the central nervous and peripheral nervous system. Neuronal substance P is stored in vesicle and is released when it	vegetables, especially as dark green leafy vegetables, milk, nuts and whole grain	their health provider before supplementing with magnesium

	comes into contact with Leukotrienes Prostaglandings histamine NDMA is a pain carrying transmitter		
Oleuropein (in olive oil)	Destroys the outer coating of bacteria, and insects destroying them in the process. It is antispasmo	Just add to salads	Helps address constipation

	dic in action and is therefore useful for IBS		
Red wine, dark chocolate, cinnamon, nutmeg, yellow mustard oil,	Anti-inflammatory in action	Just add liberally to food	Red wine will deplete some thiamine
The flavonoid Agipenin	Inhibits glutamate which is a pain carrying neurotransmitter (brain chemical)	Found in parsley, celery and many herbs	
Alpha	Useful as it	Follow	Excellent

lipoic acid	can travel anywhere as it is both water and fat soluble. It helps glutamate transport proteins which help reduce extra cellular glutamate. Extra cellular glutamate is toxic to neurons and can cause cell death.	recommenda tions on the supplement container	all round pain reliever and useful for alleviating damage in the central nervous system.
Bromelai n and aloe polyphe nols Red wine	Work on bradykinin which causes pain and inflammatio n when there are	Eat as part of a regular diet	Red wine and green tea will deplete thiamine

and green tea	microscopic tears in muscle.		

D phenylalanine	Inhibits encephalin degradation. Encephalins help prevent the transmission of pain. Morphine works on the same opioid receptor as D phenylalanine	1500-2500mg of pain	Found in many animal protein rich foods like eggs, milk meat
Fasting	Inhibits pain transmitted by neural circuits		

tryptophan	Precursor to serotonin. Inhibits pain signals and sleep latency successfully. Very useful to have in as a catch all analgesic	500mg 3 x daily	Found in poultry especially turkey breast, lentils, milk, tuna.

Please note that PPI's and diuretics are quite able to prevent absorption of nutrients required to deal with

pain or flush them immediately out of the body. Diuretics for example will flush out thiamine and magnesium and potassium, among other nutrients leading to chronic and intractable pain.

The indiscriminate use of PPI's and diuretics is concerning given that they will reduce the quality of life as well as shorten life itself.

A note from the author

Thank you for purchasing this book. Every time a book is purchased, a donation is made to one of the charities I am currently supporting.

These can be found on my author's website. See below.

Other Health Related Books by the Author

- **The Reluctant Bowel**

- A Weighty Issue
- Sleep, Perchance to Dream
- The Journey: EDS and chronic pain
- The MND diet: using nutrition to slow down the progress of neurodegeneration
- A Necessary Sorrow
- Taking another Road: Pain: its causes and what can be done about it
- The Psoriasis Diet
- The Anti Virus Diet -
- The Lipoedema Diet
- The Alzheimer's and Vascular Dementia Disease Diet.
- The Metabolic Syndrome Diet
- The EDS and Hypermobility Syndrome Diet
- Successful Aging
- Gastroparesis

And many others

These can be found here on the author's page

https://www.amazon.co.uk/-/e/B07BPQZ5CD

You may also be interested in the semi-autobiographical trilogy of the authors life found in these three books

- The Prejudged
- Where the Blackbird Never Sings
- A Summer's Symphony

And the author's children's books

- Fanny and Victorian Jack
- Fanny and the Gamekeeper's Cottage